AB POSITIVE BLOOD TYPE DIET

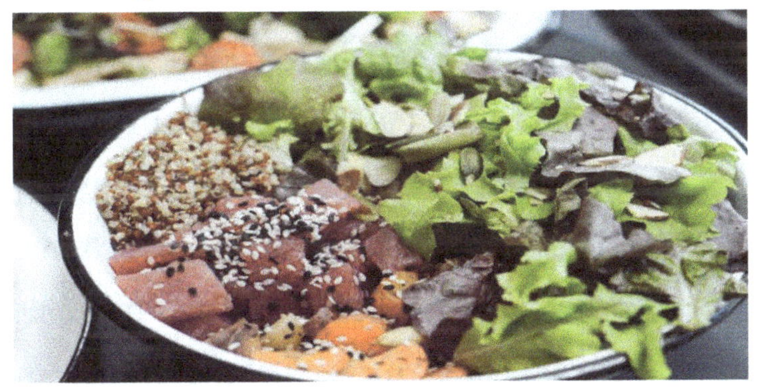

A Comprehensive Guide to Blood Type Nutrition

Linda M. Craig

Copyright © [2024] [Linda M. Craig]

Table of content

Introduction

Understanding Your AB Positive Blood Type

The AB positive blood type is a fascinating subject, rich with history, science, and implications for personal health. As the rarest of the eight basic blood types, AB positive is unique in many ways. Here's a detailed exploration of what it means to have this blood type:

Genetic Rarity and Inheritance

AB positive blood type is a result of the combination of alleles from both A and B blood types. This rarity is due to the lower odds of inheriting both an A and a B gene from one's parents. The presence of both A and B antigens on the surface of red blood cells defines this blood type, making it distinct and uncommon.

Universal Recipient

Individuals with AB positive blood are known as universal recipients in the context of red blood cell transfusions. This means they can receive red blood cells from any other blood type without the risk of an adverse reaction, thanks to the presence of both A and B antigens on their red blood cells.

Plasma Donation

While AB positive individuals can receive red blood cells from any type, they are also considered universal plasma donors. Their plasma can be given to patients of any other blood type, which is a critical component in medical treatments and emergency interventions.

Personality Traits

Some cultures, particularly in Asia, believe that blood types can influence personality traits. For AB positive individuals, they are often seen as adaptable, intelligent, and creative. However, they may also be perceived as unpredictable, indecisive.

Health Implications

The AB blood type diet theory suggests that people with AB positive blood may benefit from a diet that is a mix of the recommendations for types A and B. This includes a variety of meats, seafood, dairy, and plant-based foods, tailored to the unique digestive and immune system characteristics of the AB blood type.

Compatibility and Challenges

In terms of compatibility, AB positive individuals can face challenges due to the rarity of their blood type. In situations requiring blood transfusions, while they can receive from any type, finding AB positive donors for plasma can be more difficult due to its scarcity[2].

Understanding your AB positive blood type is more than just knowing a fact about yourself; it's about recognizing the unique aspects of your genetic makeup that can influence various areas of your life, from health to personality. Embracing this knowledge can lead to a more personalized approach to diet, lifestyle, and medical care, ensuring that you live your life to the fullest, in harmony with your biological blueprint.

The Importance of Diet for Blood Type AB

For individuals with AB positive blood type, the intersection of genetics and nutrition opens a unique dietary path that may influence health and well-being. The AB positive blood type diet is rooted in the concept that the presence of both A and B antigens in the blood affects digestion and disease susceptibility[1]. While scientific evidence supporting the diet's efficacy is limited, the idea is to optimize health by consuming foods compatible with the AB+ blood type.

Optimal Digestion and Nutrient Absorption

The diet promotes efficient digestion and absorption of nutrients, which is crucial for maintaining energy levels and overall health. For AB positive individuals, this means incorporating a mix of foods suitable for both A and B blood types, such as tofu, seafood, and green vegetables.

Energy and Immune System Support

Following the AB positive blood type diet can lead to increased energy levels and a stronger immune system. This is particularly important for AB positive individuals, who may benefit from a varied intake of foods, making the diet more sustainable than restrictive diets.

Reducing Chronic Disease Risks

The diet aims to reduce the risk of chronic diseases by tailoring food choices to the AB+ blood type. It suggests a varied intake of foods, which can be more sustainable and enjoyable than highly restrictive diets.

Personalized Health Approach

While the scientific community remains skeptical due to a lack of empirical evidence, anecdotal reports suggest that some people with AB positive blood type feel better when following this diet. This subjective experience highlights the importance of a personalized approach to health and nutrition.

Lifestyle Integration

The AB positive blood type diet doesn't specifically emphasize exercise, but a balanced lifestyle that includes physical activity is generally recommended for overall health. Smaller, frequent meals may also be digested more efficiently for those with AB positive blood type, due to lower stomach acid levels.

In conclusion, while the AB positive blood type diet lacks robust scientific validation, its focus on healthy, varied food choices may offer benefits. It's essential to consult with healthcare professionals before making significant changes to your diet or lifestyle. The importance of diet for blood type AB lies not just in the potential health benefits, but also in the journey towards a more personalized and conscious approach to eating and living.

Overview of the AB Positive Blood Type Diet

The AB Positive Blood Type Diet is a nutritional framework designed for individuals with the AB+ blood type. It's based on the premise that the food you eat reacts chemically with your blood type, and that eating a diet tailored to your blood type can help you achieve better health and prevent diseases.

Key Principles of the AB Positive Blood Type Diet:

- Food Compatibility: The diet suggests that AB+ individuals should consume foods that are compatible with both A and B blood types, such as tofu, seafood, and green vegetables

- Dietary Variety: It emphasizes a varied intake of foods, which can be more sustainable than restrictive diets.

- Chronic Disease Prevention: The goal is to optimize health by reducing the risk of chronic diseases through tailored dietary choices

How It Works:

- Genetic Considerations: The diet takes into account the genetic makeup of AB+ individuals, proposing that certain foods can enhance digestion and nutrient absorption.

- Immune System Support: It aims to boost the immune system and increase energy levels by providing a balanced mix of nutrients suitable for the AB+ blood type.

- Weight Management: While the diet claims to promote weight loss by tailoring food choices to your blood type, these claims are not backed by scientific evidence.

Starting the Diet:

- Meal Frequency: Smaller, frequent meals are recommended to be digested more efficiently due to lower stomach acid levels in AB+ individuals.

- Protein Intake: The diet advises 2-3 servings of protein per day, including options like tofu, seafood, and yogurt.

- Grains and Dairy: It includes 3-4 servings of grains daily and 2 servings of dairy, with choices like rice, oats, goat milk, and feta cheese.

Scientific Skepticism:
- Despite its popularity, the AB Positive Blood Type Diet lacks robust scientific validation. No peer-reviewed studies conclusively prove that this diet achieves its stated goals, and the scientific community remains skeptical due to a lack of empirical evidence.
- Anecdotal evidence suggests that some people feel better on the diet, but this is subjective and not supported by rigorous scientific evidence[1].

In summary, the AB Positive Blood Type Diet is a dietary approach that encourages a mix of foods suitable for both A and B blood types, with the aim of improving health and preventing chronic diseases.

Chapter One: The Science Behind Blood Type Diets

The Genetic Link to Nutrition

The field of nutrigenomics is a cutting-edge area of science that explores the intricate relationship between our genes and the foods we eat. It's a domain where genetics and nutrition intersect, revealing how our individual genetic makeup can influence our nutritional needs and health outcomes.

Understanding Nutrigenomics

Nutrigenomics examines how different genes interact with various nutrients at the molecular level. This interaction can affect everything from how we metabolize certain foods to our risk of developing specific diseases. For example, gene variants can predict how an individual's body will respond to carbohydrates and fats, potentially leading to conditions like type 2 diabetes or obesity if not managed properly.

Personalized Diets Based on Genetics

The ultimate goal of nutrigenomics is to develop personalized dietary recommendations that align with each person's genetic profile. By understanding the genetic factors that impact nutritional requirements, such as absorption, metabolism, and enzyme digestion, we can tailor diets to prevent or mitigate symptoms of existing diseases and reduce the risk of future health issue.

Gene-Diet Interactions

Certain gene polymorphisms can influence how our bodies process macronutrients. For instance, variations in the ADRB2 gene, which encodes the β2-adrenergic receptor, can affect the rate at which carbohydrates are metabolized, influencing energy balance and weight management. Similarly, the PPARG gene, which regulates lipid and carbohydrate metabolism, can have variants that impact insulin sensitivity and glucose utilization.

Challenges and Controversies

While the potential benefits of nutrigenomics are vast, there are challenges and controversies in translating this science into practice. The complexity of gene-nutrient interactions and the variability among individuals mean that creating universally effective dietary guidelines is difficult. Moreover, ethical considerations regarding genetic testing and privacy must be addressed as the field advances.

From Research to Reality

Nutrigenomics is not just a theoretical concept; it's gradually making its way into clinical practice. As more is understood about the genetic blueprint of nutrition, healthcare providers can offer more precise nutritional advice, moving away from one-size-fits-all dietary recommendations to more customized approaches that consider an individual's unique genetic makeup.

In summary, the genetic link to nutrition is a profound discovery that has the potential to revolutionize the way we think about food and health. By embracing the principles of nutrigenomics, we can look forward to a future where our diets are as unique as our DNA, offering us the best chance at a healthy life.

Blood Type and Digestive Chemistry

The concept of blood type and digestive chemistry is rooted in the idea that the type of blood flowing through our veins can influence our digestive processes. This notion is part of the blood type diet hypothesis, which suggests that people with different blood types may digest and react to food differently due to the specific antigens present on their red blood cells.

ABO Blood Types and Carbohydrate Chemistry

The ABO blood group system is the most recognized classification of blood types, named after the antigens found on the surface of red blood cells. These antigens are essentially chains of carbohydrates, or sugars, that vary slightly between the A, B, and O blood types. The presence of these antigens can theoretically affect the body's immune response to certain foods.

Digestive Enzymes and Blood Types

The digestive system is equipped with a variety of enzymes that break down food into nutrients. The theory posits that blood types may influence the secretion levels and activity of these digestive enzymes. For instance, individuals with type AB blood might have a combination of characteristics from both type A (higher levels of certain digestive enzymes) and type B (different immune responses to certain foods).

Gut Microbiota and Blood Type

Recent research has also explored the relationship between blood type and the gut microbiota—the vast community of microorganisms living in our digestive tracts. These microbes play a crucial role in digestion, and there is emerging evidence that blood type antigens can influence the composition of the gut microbiota, potentially affecting digestive health.

Nutrient Absorption and Blood Type

The absorption of nutrients in the small intestine might also be affected by blood type. Specific transporters and receptors that facilitate nutrient uptake could vary in efficiency depending on one's blood type, although this area of research is still in its infancy and requires further investigation.

Scientific Considerations

While the blood type diet has gained popularity, it's important to note that the scientific community has not reached a consensus on the validity of the blood type and digestive chemistry connection. Most studies have not found conclusive evidence to support the idea that blood type significantly influences digestion or diet.

In conclusion, the relationship between blood type and digestive chemistry is a fascinating topic that combines immunology, genetics, and nutrition. While intriguing, the blood type diet remains a hypothesis that lacks robust scientific validation.

The Immune System and Blood Type AB

The immune system is a complex network of cells, tissues, and organs that work together to defend the body against infections and diseases. Blood type AB, with its unique combination of A and B antigens, interacts with the immune system in several ways that are worth exploring.

Antigens and Antibodies

Individuals with blood type AB have both A and B antigens on the surface of their red blood cells. These antigens are part of the body's natural defense system and can influence the immune response. Unlike other blood types, AB does not produce anti-A or anti-B antibodies, which means they can accept red blood cells from any other blood type during transfusions.

Immune Response

The immune system recognizes and responds to antigens as a normal part of its function. For blood type AB, the presence of both A and B antigens means that the immune system is accustomed to a wider variety of antigens, which could theoretically lead to a more tolerant immune response when exposed to different blood types.

Autoimmune Diseases

Research has suggested that certain blood types may be more prone to specific autoimmune diseases, where the immune system mistakenly attacks the body's own tissues. However, the evidence linking blood type AB to specific autoimmune conditions is inconsistent and requires further study.

Transfusion and Organ Transplantation

Blood type AB individuals are considered universal recipients for plasma transfusions because they do not have anti-A or anti-B antibodies. This makes them less likely to reject transfused blood. However, when it comes to organ transplantation, compatibility is more complex and involves additional factors beyond blood type.

Infection Susceptibility

Some studies have investigated whether blood type AB might be associated with an increased susceptibility to certain infections, but the results are not conclusive. The immune system's ability to fight off infections is influenced by many factors, including genetics, environment, and overall health.

Nutrition and Immunity

The blood type diet hypothesis extends to the immune system, suggesting that people with blood type AB might benefit from a diet that supports their unique antigen profile. However, this concept remains controversial and is not widely accepted in the scientific community due to a lack of empirical evidence.

In summary, while blood type AB has certain characteristics that can interact with the immune system, the full extent of these interactions and their implications for health are not fully understood.

Chapter Two: Optimal Foods for AB Positive

Beneficial Meats and Seafood

For individuals with blood type AB positive, the diet is often characterized by a focus on balance between meats and plant-based foods. The AB positive blood type diet suggests a mix of foods suitable for both A and B blood types, emphasizing tofu, seafood, and green vegetables.

Beneficial Meats for Blood Type AB Positive:

- Turkey: A lean source of protein that is easier to digest for AB positive individuals compared to red meat.

- Lamb: Often recommended for its richness in essential amino acids and compatibility with AB blood type.
- Rabbit: A lean meat that is considered beneficial for its low-fat content and high protein quality.

Beneficial Seafood for Blood Type AB Positive:
- Salmon: Rich in omega-3 fatty acids, which are important for cardiovascular health and cognitive function.
- Cod: A good source of lean protein and vitamin B12, which is essential for nerve health and energy production.
- Mackerel: Another excellent source of omega-3 fatty acids, as well as protein and selenium.

Additional Seafood Options:

- Grouper: Known for its mild flavor and firm texture, grouper is a versatile seafood option for AB positive individuals.

- Snapper: Provides a good balance of flavor and nutrition, offering protein and essential vitamins and minerals.

- Mahi Mahi: A tropical fish that is both flavorful and beneficial for its protein content and heart-healthy fats.

Dairy and Eggs: Selecting the Best Options

For individuals with blood type AB positive, selecting the right dairy and eggs is an important aspect of following the blood type diet. The diet suggests that certain dairy products and eggs can be beneficial, while others may not be as compatible with this blood type.

Beneficial Dairy Products for Blood Type AB Positive:

- Cottage Cheese: A versatile dairy product that is easy to digest and can be included in various recipes.

- Farmer's Cheese: Similar to cottage cheese, farmer's cheese is gentle on the stomach and rich in protein.

- Feta Cheese: Made from sheep's milk, feta is considered beneficial for its probiotic content and easier digestibility.

- Goat Cheese and Goat Milk: Goat milk products are often recommended for AB positive individuals due to their lower lactose content.

- Kefir: A fermented milk drink that contains beneficial bacteria, kefir is known for its probiotic properties.

- Mozzarella: This cheese is typically well-tolerated and can be a good source of calcium.

- Ricotta: A soft cheese that is lower in fat and can be a part of a healthy diet for AB positive individuals.

- Yogurt: Especially yogurts with live cultures, as they can aid in digestion and support gut health.

Eggs:

Eggs are generally considered neutral for blood type AB positive. They can be a part of the diet in moderation, providing a good source of protein and other nutrients.

Dairy and Eggs to Avoid for Blood Type AB Positive:

- American Cheese: Highly processed and often contains additives that may not be beneficial for AB positive individuals.

- Blue Cheese: The mold used in blue cheese can sometimes cause adverse reactions.

- Brie and Camembert: These soft cheeses may not be as easily digested by those with AB positive blood.

- Butter and Buttermilk: High in saturated fat, these may be less suitable for AB positive individuals.

- Whole Cow's Milk: The higher fat content and lactose levels may make cow's milk less ideal.

- Ice Cream: Often high in sugar and fat, ice cream is best consumed in limited amounts.

- Parmesan and Provolone: These aged cheeses may be harder to digest for some AB positive individuals.

Vegetables and Fruits for AB Positive

For those with blood type AB positive, the diet is often characterized by a balance between plant-based foods and select animal proteins. When it comes to vegetables and fruits, certain types are considered particularly beneficial for this blood type.

Beneficial Vegetables for Blood Type AB Positive:

- Beet Greens: Rich in iron and beneficial for blood health.

- Broccoli: Contains sulforaphane, which has been shown to have anti-cancer properties.

- Cauliflower: A versatile vegetable that can be used in various dishes, providing fiber and vitamins.

- Celery: Low in calories and high in water content, making it a hydrating choice.
- Cucumber: Another hydrating vegetable that's also good for skin health.
- Garlic: Known for its immune-boosting properties.
- Kale: A nutrient-dense leafy green, high in vitamins A, C, and K.
- Parsnips: A good source of fiber and folate.
- Sweet Potatoes: Rich in beta-carotene and complex carbohydrates.
- Yams: Similar to sweet potatoes, yams are a good source of fiber and vitamin C.

Vegetables to Avoid for Blood Type AB Positive:

- Artichokes: May not be as easily digested by those with AB positive blood.
- Corn: Can affect insulin levels and digestion for AB positive individuals.

- Peppers: Some individuals may find peppers irritating to the stomach.

- Radishes: Can be too harsh for the digestive system of those with AB positive blood.

Beneficial Fruits for Blood Type AB Positive:

- Cherries: Can help reduce inflammation and provide antioxidants.

- Cranberries: Good for urinary tract health and also provide antioxidants.

- Figs: High in fiber and can aid in digestion.

- Grapes: Contain resveratrol, which is beneficial for heart health.

- Kiwi: A good source of vitamin C and digestive enzymes.

- Lemons: Can aid in detoxification and alkalizing the body.

- Pineapples: Contain bromelain, an enzyme that aids in digestion.

Fruits to Avoid for Blood Type AB Positive:

- Bananas: May contribute to mucus production and can be difficult to digest for some.

- Mangoes: High sugar content may not be ideal for AB positive individuals.

- Oranges: Acidic nature can lead to digestive issues for some with AB positive blood.

Chapter Three: Avoids and Alternatives

Foods to Avoid for Blood Type AB

For individuals with blood type AB positive, the blood type diet suggests that certain foods may not be as beneficial and could potentially interfere with their overall health and well-being.

Meats to Avoid:

- Beef: It may be difficult to digest and can potentially lead to stomach discomfort.
- Chicken: The muscle tissue of chicken contains a lectin that can irritate the blood and digestive tract of AB positive individuals.
- Pork: Often high in fat and may not be compatible with the digestive system of those with AB positive blood.

Seafood to Avoid:

- Barracuda: This fish can contain high levels of mercury and other toxins.

- Eel: May be too oily and not as beneficial for AB positive individuals.

- Shellfish: Including shrimp, crab, and lobster, which can be allergenic and not well tolerated.

Dairy Products to Avoid:

- American Cheese: Highly processed and may contain additives that are not beneficial.

- Blue Cheese: Contains mold that can sometimes cause adverse reactions.

- Ice Cream: Often high in sugar and fat, which is best consumed in limited amounts.

Grains to Avoid:

- Buckwheat: Can lead to a drop in insulin production for AB positive individuals.

- Corn: Can affect insulin levels and digestion, potentially leading to obesity and diabetes.

- Wheat: Contains lectins that can interfere with insulin efficiency and lead to weight gain.

Vegetables to Avoid:

- Artichokes: May not be easily digested by those with AB positive blood.

- Bell Peppers: Some individuals may find them irritating to the stomach.

- Tomatoes: Contain lectins that can lead to stomach distress for AB positive individuals.

Fruits to Avoid:

- Bananas: Can contribute to mucus production and may be difficult to digest for some.

- Mangoes: High sugar content may not be ideal for AB positive individuals.

- Oranges: Their acidic nature can lead to digestive issues for some with AB positive blood.

Nuts and Seeds to Avoid:

- Poppy Seeds: Can interfere with the metabolism of AB positive individuals.

- Sesame Seeds: May irritate the stomach and lead to adverse reactions.

- Sunflower Seeds: Can affect the digestive tract negatively.

Beverages to Avoid:

- Alcohol: Especially distilled liquor, can be harsh on the stomach lining.

- Coffee: Can increase stomach acid and lead to digestive discomfort.

- Soda: High in sugar and chemicals, which can disrupt the digestive system.

Healthy Substitutes for Common Allergens

For individuals with blood type AB positive, finding healthy substitutes for common allergens can be an important part of maintaining a balanced diet. Here's a detailed guide on alternative options that are more compatible with the AB positive blood type diet:

Substitutes for Wheat and Gluten:

- Rice: A versatile grain that can be used in place of wheat in many recipes.

- Quinoa: A protein-rich seed that serves as a great gluten-free alternative to wheat-based grains.

- Oats: Ensure they are labeled gluten-free to avoid cross-contamination with wheat.

Substitutes for Cow's Milk:

- Goat Milk: Often better tolerated by those with AB positive blood type and can be used in place of cow's milk.
- Almond Milk: A dairy-free alternative that's rich in vitamins and minerals.
- Coconut Milk: Suitable for cooking and baking, adding a creamy texture without dairy.

Substitutes for Corn:

- Millet: A gluten-free grain that can replace corn in recipes.
- Amaranth: Another gluten-free option that can be used as a substitute for cornmeal.

Substitutes for Peanuts:

- Almonds: Can be used in place of peanuts for snacking or in recipes.

- Sunflower Seeds: A good alternative for those allergic to peanuts, and can be used to make sunflower seed butter.

Substitutes for Soy:
- Tempeh: Made from fermented soybeans, tempeh is often better tolerated than other soy products.
- Chickpeas: Can be used to make hummus, a great substitute for soy-based dips.

Substitutes for Shellfish:
- White Fish: Such as cod or tilapia, can be used as a substitute for shellfish in recipes.
- Imitation Crab: Made from fish, it can be a suitable alternative for those who are allergic to shellfish.

Substitutes for Eggs:

- Chia Seeds: When mixed with water, chia seeds form a gel that can replace eggs in baking.
- Flaxseeds: Similar to chia, flaxseeds can be used as an egg substitute in recipes.

Substitutes for Tomatoes:

- Roasted Red Peppers: Can be pureed to make a tomato-free sauce.
- Beets: Offer a similar color and can be used in some recipes as a tomato substitute.

Managing Cravings and Making Smart Choices

Managing cravings and making smart dietary choices can be a challenge, especially when following a specific diet like the one for blood type AB positive. Here's a guide to help you navigate through cravings and maintain a balanced diet:

Understanding Cravings:

- Identify Triggers: Recognize what triggers your cravings. It could be emotional, such as stress or boredom, or physical, like hunger or nutrient deficiencies.
- Mindful Eating: Practice being present while eating. Enjoy the flavors, textures, and sensations of your food, which can help reduce overeating and satisfy cravings.

Smart Dietary Choices for Blood Type AB Positive:

- Balanced Meals: Ensure each meal includes a balance of proteins, carbohydrates, and fats to keep blood sugar levels stable and reduce cravings[1].

- Frequent Small Meals: Eating smaller, more frequent meals can help manage hunger and prevent intense cravings.

- Hydration: Sometimes, thirst is mistaken for hunger. Stay hydrated to help curb unnecessary snacking.

Substituting Cravings:

- Healthy Alternatives: Find healthier alternatives that satisfy your cravings. For sweet cravings, opt for fruits like cherries or grapes. For salty cravings, try lightly salted nuts or seeds.

- Portion Control: If you indulge in a craving, do so in moderation. Have a small portion of what you're craving and savor it.

Planning Ahead:

- Meal Prep: Prepare meals and snacks in advance to avoid impulsive eating decisions.

- Grocery List: Stick to a shopping list based on your blood type AB positive diet to avoid buying tempting foods that are not beneficial for your blood type.

Emotional Support:

- Stress Management: Engage in activities that reduce stress, such as exercise, meditation, or hobbies, to prevent emotional eating.
- Support Network: Build a support network of friends or family who understand your dietary goals and can offer encouragement.

Long-Term Sustainability:

- Flexible Approach: Allow yourself occasional treats to avoid feeling deprived, which can lead to binge eating.
- Lifestyle Integration: Incorporate your diet into your lifestyle in a way that feels natural and sustainable.

Chapter Four: Meal Planning and Recipes

Crafting a Weekly Meal Plan

Crafting a weekly meal plan tailored to the AB positive blood type involves incorporating a variety of foods that are beneficial for this blood group, while also ensuring a balanced intake of nutrients. Here's a detailed guide to help you create a weekly meal plan:

Day 1:

- Breakfast: Scrambled eggs with spinach and feta cheese.

- Lunch: Grilled salmon salad with mixed greens, cherry tomatoes, and a lemon-olive oil dressing.

- Dinner: Turkey stir-fry with broccoli, bell peppers, and quinoa.

Day 2:

- Breakfast:Greek yogurt with sliced kiwi and a drizzle of honey.
- Lunch: Lentil soup with a side of mixed greens and goat cheese.
- Dinner: Baked cod with roasted sweet potatoes and steamed kale.

Day 3:

- Breakfast: Smoothie with almond milk, banana, and a scoop of protein powder.
- Lunch: Tofu and vegetable curry with brown rice.
- Dinner: Lamb chops with a side of roasted cauliflower and a cucumber salad.

Day 4:

- Breakfast: Oatmeal topped with blueberries and a sprinkle of chia seeds.

- Lunch: Turkey and avocado wrap with whole grain tortilla and a side of carrot sticks.

- Dinner: Grilled mackerel with a side of sautéed beet greens and quinoa.

Day 5:

- Breakfast: Cottage cheese with sliced peaches and almonds.

- Lunch: Quinoa salad with grilled vegetables and a tahini dressing.

- Dinner: Stir-fried tempeh with broccoli, carrots, and brown rice.

Day 6:

- Breakfast: Kefir with granola and fresh berries.

- Lunch: Tuna salad with mixed greens, cucumbers, and olives.

- Dinner: Roast lamb with parsnips and a side of green beans.

Day 7:

- Breakfast: Poached eggs on a bed of arugula with gluten-free toast.

- Lunch: Chickpea and vegetable stew with a side of brown rice.

- Dinner: Grilled mahi-mahi with a side of roasted Brussels sprouts and a sweet potato mash.

Snacks:

- Fresh fruits like cherries, cranberries, and pineapple.

- Nuts such as almonds and walnuts.

- Vegetables sticks with hummus.

Beverages:

- Plenty of water throughout the day.

- Herbal teas like green tea or chamomile.

- Freshly squeezed fruit juices in moderation.

This meal plan includes a variety of foods that are considered beneficial for the AB positive blood type, such as tofu, seafood, and green vegetables[123]. It's designed to provide a balanced mix of protein, carbohydrates, and fats, along with essential vitamins and minerals. Remember to adjust portion sizes and food choices based on individual nutritional needs and preferences.

Creating recipes for individuals with blood type AB positive involves selecting ingredients that are beneficial and avoiding those that are not recommended for this blood type. Here are some recipes for breakfast, lunch, and dinner that align with the AB positive blood type diet:

Breakfast: Mediterranean Tofu Scramble

- Ingredients:

  - 1/2 block firm tofu, crumbled

  - 1/4 cup diced tomatoes

  - 1/4 cup chopped spinach

  - 1/4 cup chopped olives

  - 1/4 cup crumbled feta cheese

  - 1 tbsp olive oil

  - Salt and pepper to taste

  - Fresh herbs (basil or parsley) for garnish

- Instructions:

1. Heat olive oil in a pan over medium heat.

2. Add crumbled tofu and cook until slightly golden.

3. Stir in tomatoes, spinach, and olives, and cook for another 2-3 minutes.

4. Season with salt and pepper.

5. Just before serving, mix in the feta cheese and garnish with fresh herbs.

Lunch: Grilled Salmon and Quinoa Salad

- Ingredients:

- 1 salmon fillet
- 1 cup cooked quinoa
- 1/2 cup diced cucumber
- 1/2 cup cherry tomatoes, halved
- 1/4 cup chopped red onion
- 2 tbsp lemon juice
- 2 tbsp olive oil
- Salt and pepper to taste
- Mixed greens for serving

- Instructions:

1. Grill the salmon fillet until cooked to your preference.

2. In a bowl, combine quinoa, cucumber, cherry tomatoes, and red onion.

3. Whisk together lemon juice, olive oil, salt, and pepper to create a dressing.

4. Toss the quinoa salad with the dressing.

5. Serve the grilled salmon on a bed of mixed greens, topped with the quinoa salad.

Dinner: Turkey and Vegetable Stir-Fry

- Ingredients:

- 1/2 lb turkey breast, thinly sliced
- 1 cup broccoli florets
- 1/2 cup sliced carrots
- 1/2 cup bell pepper strips
- 2 cloves garlic, minced
- 1 tbsp soy sauce (or tamari for gluten-free option)
- 1 tbsp sesame oil

- 1 tsp ginger, grated

- Brown rice or rice noodles for serving

- Instructions:

1. Heat sesame oil in a wok or large pan over high heat.

2. Add turkey slices and stir-fry until browned.

3. Add garlic, ginger, broccoli, carrots, and bell peppers. Stir-fry until vegetables are tender-crisp.

4. Pour in soy sauce and toss everything to coat evenly.

5. Serve hot over brown rice or rice noodles.

These recipes incorporate foods that are considered beneficial for blood type AB positive, such as tofu, seafood, and turkey, while avoiding those that are not recommended, like chicken and beef.

Snacks and Beverages: Tasty and Healthy Ideas

For individuals with blood type AB positive, choosing snacks and beverages that align with their dietary needs is essential for maintaining overall health. Here's a guide to tasty and healthy snack and beverage ideas suitable for the AB positive blood type diet:

Snacks:

- Fruits: Opt for fruits like cherries, grapes, figs, and pineapple, which are considered beneficial for AB positive individuals. These fruits not only satisfy sweet cravings but also provide essential vitamins and antioxidants.
- Nuts and Seeds: Almonds and walnuts are good options for a quick, protein-rich snack. They offer healthy fats and can help keep you full between meals.

- Cheese: Small portions of cheeses like mozzarella, ricotta, or goat cheese can be a satisfying snack and provide a good source of calcium.

- Vegetable Sticks: Carrot, celery, and cucumber sticks paired with hummus or a yogurt-based dip are both refreshing and nutritious.

- Tofu: Marinated tofu cubes can be a savory snack that's high in protein and aligns with the AB positive dietary recommendations.

Beverages:

- Green Tea: A great alternative to coffee, green tea offers a gentle caffeine boost along with antioxidants.

- Herbal Teas: Chamomile, peppermint, or ginger tea can be soothing and support digestion.

- Water: Staying hydrated is crucial. Infuse water with slices of lemon, cucumber, or berries for added flavor.

- Juices: Freshly squeezed fruit juices, particularly from beneficial fruits, can be enjoyed in moderation. Be mindful of the sugar content and opt for juices without added sugars.

- Kefir: This fermented milk beverage is a good source of probiotics and can support gut health.

When selecting snacks and beverages, it's important to listen to your body's signals and choose items that satisfy your cravings while providing nutritional benefits. Remember, the key is balance and moderation.

Chapter Five: Lifestyle Adjustments for AB Positive

Exercise Recommendations for AB Positive

Exercise recommendations for individuals with AB positive blood type can be quite unique due to the mixed nature of their blood type, which combines characteristics from both Type A and Type B. Here's a detailed guide:

Exercise Recommendations for AB Positive Blood Type

1. Balance of Intensity:

   - Type A Characteristics: Individuals with Type A elements may experience muscle and joint stiffness, so high-impact cardio activities might not be ideal.

- Type B Characteristics: Those with Type B traits tend to have high energy levels and can benefit from exercises that help burn off surplus energy.

2. Recommended Activities:

- Fluid Exercises: Activities like yoga and tai chi are recommended as they can help AB types to be more emotionally stable.

- Aerobic Exercise: Aerobic exercises are preferred to maintain manageable baseline stress levels.

3. Combining Exercise Types:

- The ideal exercise regimen for an AB combines activities suitable for both Type A and Type B blood types.

4. Frequency and Duration:

- Regular exercise is a must. It's recommended to engage in physical activity several times a week, with a mix of both calming and energetic exercises.

5. Emotional Considerations:

- Type ABs tend to bottle up emotions, so exercises that also provide emotional release and stability are beneficia.l

6. Personalization:

- It's important to listen to your body and adjust the intensity and type of exercise according to how you feel on any given day.

Stress Management Techniques

Understanding Stress and Blood Type AB+

Blood type AB+ individuals may have unique physiological responses to stress. While there is no direct scientific evidence linking blood types to specific stress management strategies, it's important to consider a holistic approach that addresses both physical and emotional well-being.

Physical Activity

Engaging in regular physical activity is beneficial for everyone, including those with blood type AB+. Activities such as walking, swimming, biking, or jogging can help release tension in the body and improve mood.

Diet and Substance Use

Maintaining a balanced diet and avoiding overeating are crucial. Limiting alcohol intake and refraining from smoking can also help manage stress levels effectively

Time Management

Good time management can reduce stress significantly. Allow yourself enough time to complete tasks without rushing. Learn to say "no" and avoid overcommitting to reduce the amount of tension in your life.

Emotional Control

Recognize what you can and cannot control. Accepting things you cannot change and focusing on how you handle them emotionally can reduce stress. Techniques like meditation, progressive muscle relaxation, guided imagery, deep breathing exercises, and yoga can be particularly helpful.

Social Support

Strengthening your social network by connecting with others through classes, organizations, or support groups can provide emotional support and reduce stress.

Professional Help

If stress becomes overwhelming, it may lead to anxiety disorders. It's important to discuss any stress or anxiety issues with a healthcare professional to learn better management techniques.

Remember, stress management is not one-size-fits-all, and what works for one person may not work for another. It's about finding the right balance and techniques that work for you personally.

Long-term Health Strategies for Blood Type AB

Here's a comprehensive guide on long-term health strategies for individuals with blood type AB+:

Diet and Nutrition

- Diverse Diet: The AB+ blood type diet suggests a varied intake of foods, making it more sustainable than restrictive diets.

- Recommended Foods: Include tofu, seafood, green vegetables, and certain dairy products like yogurt and kefir.

- Foods to Avoid: It's advised to limit caffeine, alcohol, and smoked and cured meats.

Exercise

- Balanced Routine: A combination of exercises suitable for both A and B blood types is recommended, including calming exercises like yoga and tai chi.
- Regular Physical Activity: Engage in activities that promote cardiovascular health and stress reduction.

Health Screenings

- Regular Check-ups: Stay up-to-date with health screenings to monitor for conditions that may be more prevalent in individuals with AB+ blood type, such as heart disease and anemia.

Lifestyle Adjustments

- Stress Management: Implement stress-reducing practices such as meditation and deep breathing exercises

- Avoid Pollutants: Stay out of highly polluted areas and consider exercising indoors when air quality is poor.

Heart Health

- Heart-Healthy Diet: Emphasize fruits, vegetables, whole grains, fish, and nuts to maintain a heart-healthy diet.
- Life's Essential: Following the American Heart Association's guidelines can add years to your life and reduce the risk of thrombosis-related outcomes.

General Wellness

- No Smoking: Avoid smoking to reduce the risk of chronic diseases.
- Hydration: Maintain adequate hydration for overall health and well-being.

Conclusion

In conclusion, the "AB Positive Blood Type Diet" book offers a unique perspective on nutrition and wellness, tailored to those with the AB+ blood type. This book serves as a guide to understanding how certain foods and lifestyle choices can potentially harmonize with the AB+ blood type to optimize health and well-being.

The journey to health is deeply personal, and this book encourages readers to explore and discover what works best for their bodies. Whether it's incorporating more tofu and seafood into your diet, engaging in a mix of calming and cardiovascular exercises, or finding balance through stress management techniques, the key is to listen to your body and make adjustments that promote a healthier, more vibrant life.

As we close this chapter, remember that the most important takeaway is to approach your health holistically, with mindfulness and intention. The "AB Positive Blood Type Diet" is more than just a set of dietary guidelines; it's a stepping stone towards a more attuned and conscious way of living. May this book be a valuable companion on your path to wellness.

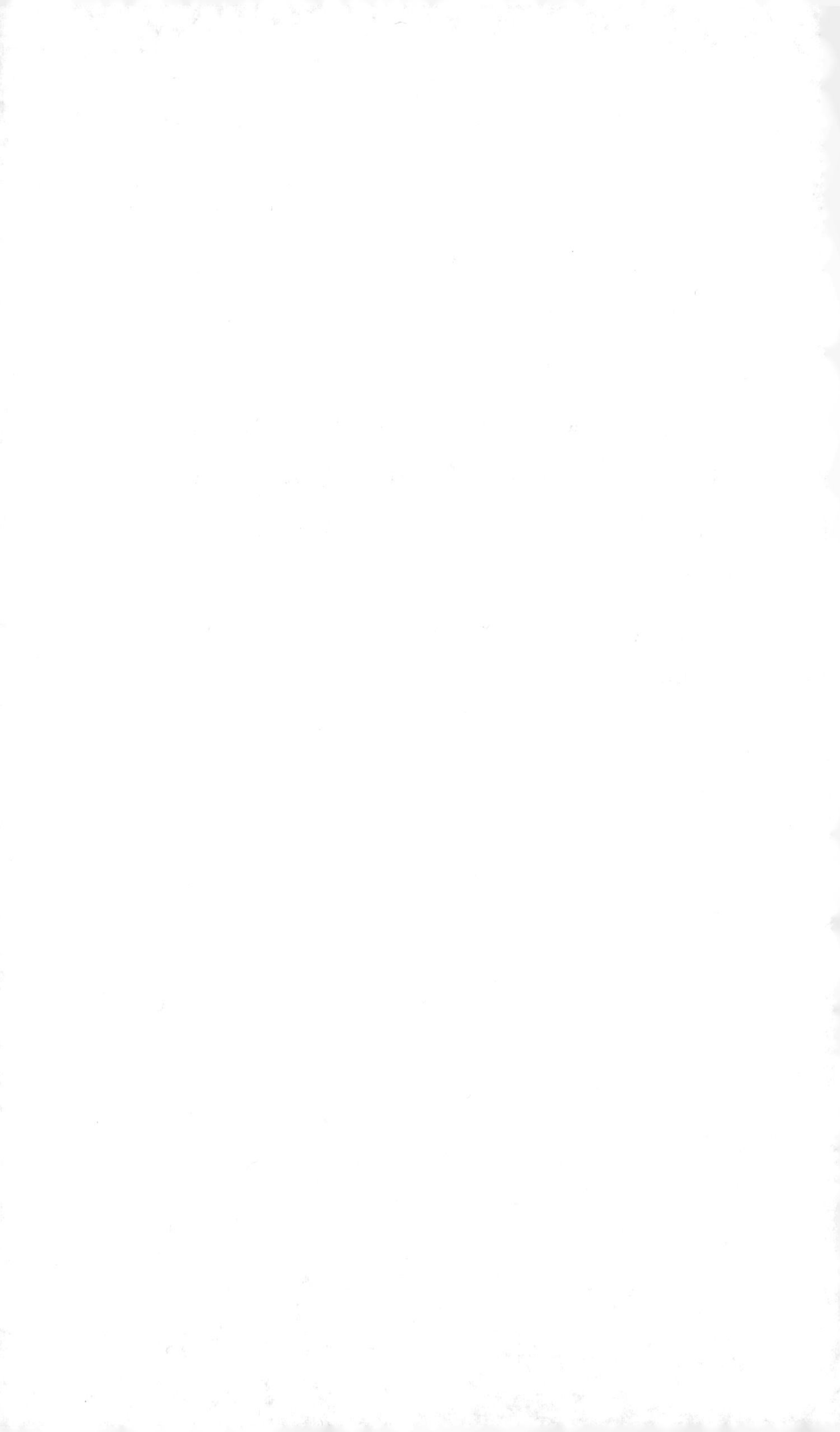

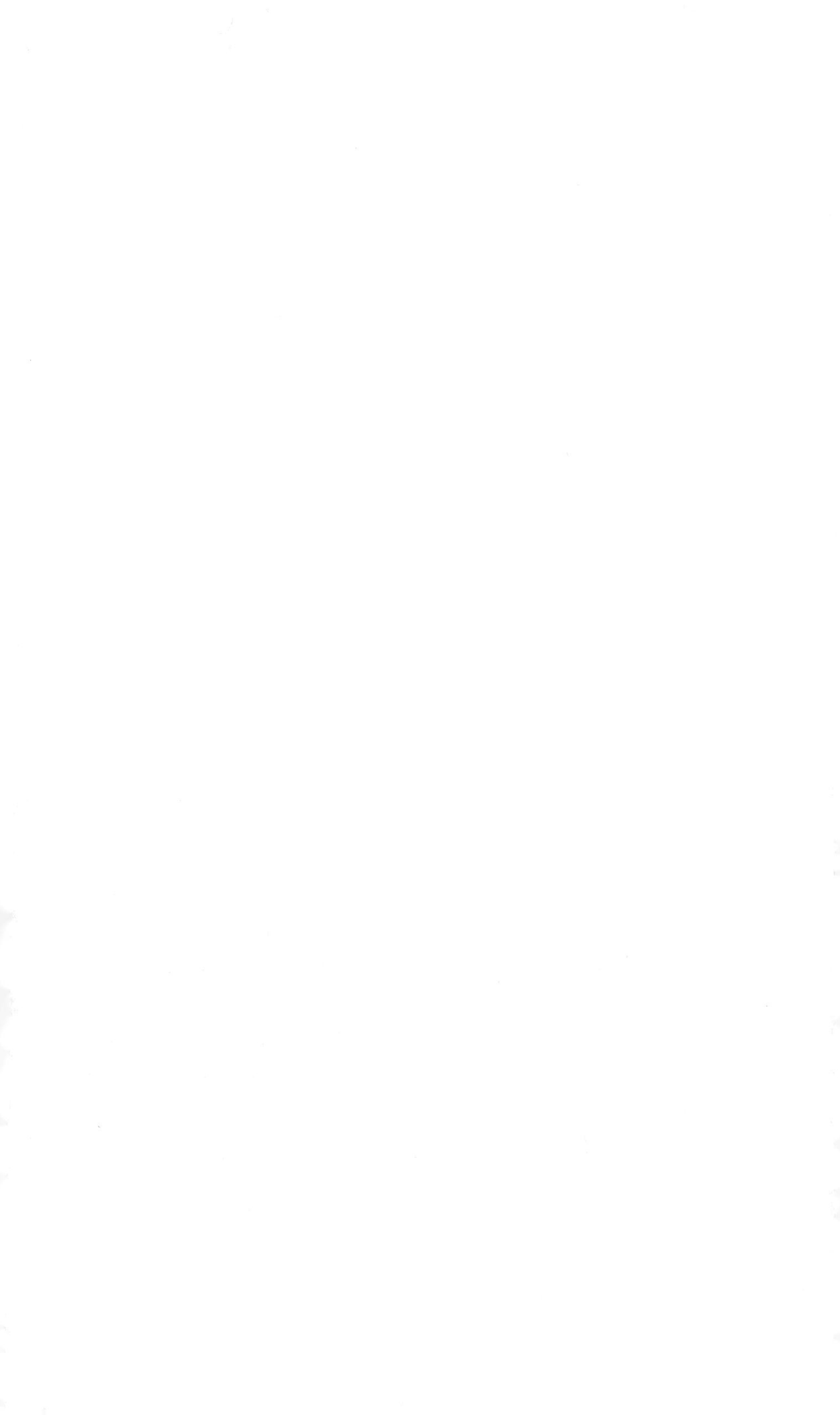

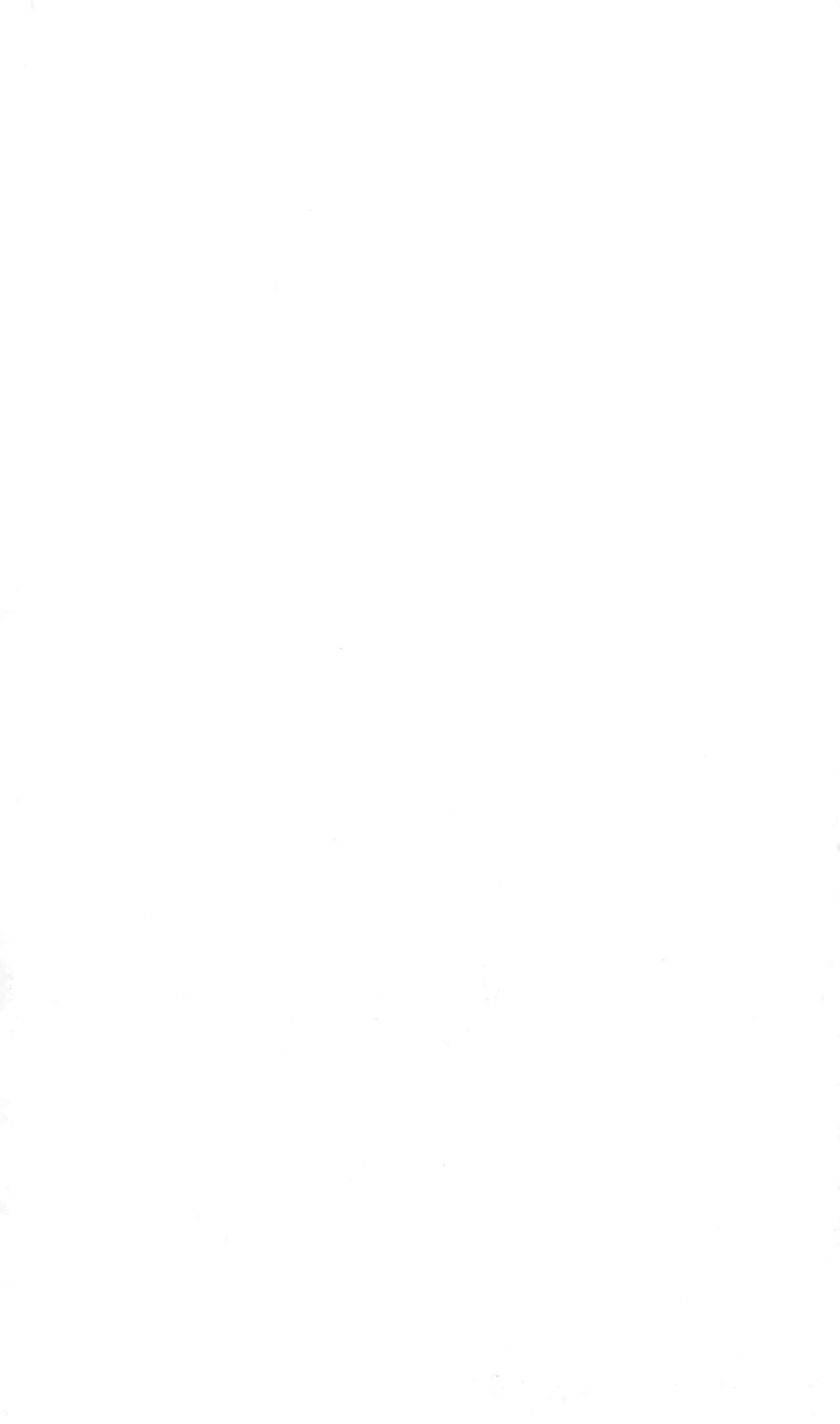